Revolutionizing Water Access Through Modern Technology: A Step Towards Global Change

Investigative Water Research Book

By Meklit Garedew Gebrewold

© 2024 by Meklit Garedew

Cover design by Meklit Garedew Gebrewold

Meklit Garedew Gebrewold's contact: meklitgara91@gmail.com

Introduction

Access to clean and safe water is a fundamental human right, and ensuring its availability can transform lives across the globe. Water is the cornerstone of health, agriculture, and overall well-being, yet millions still struggle to access it. Facilitating water access, especially in areas plagued by scarcity, can break cycles of poverty, improve public health, and elevate the quality of life for countless communities. The ripple effect of accessible water extends to education, economic development, and environmental sustainability, making it a global priority that must not be overlooked.

The United Nations plays a pivotal role in addressing global challenges, and the facilitation of water access should be at the forefront of its agenda. By allocating resources and initiating large-scale projects, the UN can drive significant progress toward ensuring that every person, regardless of location, has reliable access to clean water. This universal water supply requires cooperation and commitment from governments and UN to create sustainable, long-lasting solutions.

Moreover, as humanity looks toward future exploration and the possibility of inhabiting other planets, it is essential to consider how water can be transported and made accessible in extraterrestrial environments. This potential not only highlights the importance of innovation in water technology but also raises the need for global organizations like the UN to take proactive measures in supporting water solutions that transcend Earth.

In addition to global efforts, universities and research institutions must take an active role in addressing water scarcity. Government-funded universities, in particular, have the capacity to develop and implement innovative technologies to tackle this pressing issue. By dedicating time, resources, and research to finding practical, cost-effective solutions, these institutions can spearhead transformative change. Their involvement could lead to groundbreaking discoveries that make water more accessible, especially in regions most affected by shortages.

During my years in medical school, I initiated research on water accessibility after noticing a severe shortage in a specific region of Ethiopia, an area historically known for its water challenges. Every Ethiopian is aware of the significance of this region's long-standing struggle. Even since I was a little kid the way my parents used to manage the water supply for our family is way too unique and I do admire them in such a sincere and lovely way. I do always thank God almighty about them in the name of Jesus Christ for God has given me such awesome plus brave parents! So I was well equipped with so much great wisdoms from my parents then here I am with a priceless fruit in such unpredictable calling of God almighty on my life! Here I am with such a great investigative water research book! With proper dedication and collaboration between academic institutions, governments, and the UN, universal access to water can become a reality.

Revolutionizing Water Access Through Modern Technology: A Step Towards Global Change

Water is a fundamental necessity for all human life, and its scarcity remains a pressing challenge for millions around the world. While we have made significant advancements in various sectors of life, the issue of providing clean and accessible water for everyone still lingers in many parts of the universe. Ensuring that every person has access to adequate water resources is essential not only for survival but also for improving quality of life. Water is critical for agriculture, sanitation, industry, and daily personal use. The question is, how can we harness modern technology to facilitate water needs globally, especially in areas where it remains scarce?

A potential solution lies in utilizing underground water sources from one's own compound. With the advancement of modern machine technology, it is possible to develop equipment that can extract groundwater in a cost-effective and sustainable manner. Imagine a future where households, especially in remote or arid regions, could have personal access to water through specialized technology that taps into underground reserves. This would revolutionize how we think about water supply and usage, eliminating reliance on centralized, and often strained, water infrastructures. For regions that struggle to find surface water, this could be a game-changer.

The beauty of this approach is its ability to empower individuals and communities to take control of their water needs. By creating a small-scale, efficient machine to extract underground water, families could become self-sufficient in their water consumption, reducing the burden on over-exploited natural sources. In times of climate uncertainty, where droughts are becoming more common, this technology could provide a lifeline to families at risk of water insecurity. Furthermore, it offers a sustainable alternative to traditional methods of water sourcing, which often involve lengthy, expensive infrastructure projects that are difficult to maintain.

However, for this to work effectively, I need to ensure that the technology is widely available and accessible to all, especially in low-income areas where water scarcity is most severe. This is where the role of governments becomes crucial. Governments, in collaboration with universities and research institutions, have the capacity to develop, fund, and distribute these modern machines on a national and global scale. Government support is necessary to subsidize the technology, making it affordable for the people who need it most. Collaboration with local academic institutions would provide the technical know-how to develop these machines, creating opportunities for innovation while addressing a critical global need.

In cases where underground water is not accessible in one's own compound or region, a more creative solution is required. One such idea is the use of modern helicopters specifically manufactured to help transport water to remote areas where water wells cannot be established. These helicopters could be equipped with advanced water storage systems and function similarly to air ambulances, providing immediate water relief to those in critical need. Governments, once again, would play a pivotal role in this innovation, developing these specialized helicopters through public-private partnerships and university-driven research.

The role of international bodies such as the United Nations cannot be underestimated in addressing the global water crisis. The UN, with its global influence and resources, should prioritize facilitating water access for every individual. By partnering with nations and supporting the research, development, and deployment of modern water-extraction technologies, the UN can help ensure that everyone, regardless of their location, has access to safe and reliable water. This kind of commitment would align with the UN's Sustainable Development Goals, particularly Goal 6, which aims to ensure the availability and sustainable management of water for all.

The impact of providing water access through modern technology would be profound. It would not only save lives by reducing waterborne diseases and promoting sanitation but also create opportunities for economic growth. In agricultural communities, for example, access to consistent water supplies would enable farmers to increase productivity, ensuring food security. In urban settings, reliable water access would improve living conditions and promote hygiene, contributing to overall public health. This approach would significantly boost the well-being of populations worldwide.

Introducing water-extracting technology at a household level would democratize water access, creating a system that is not reliant on the inefficiencies of government distribution or private monopolies. It would also alleviate political tensions surrounding water rights and distribution, which are common in water-scarce regions. In many cases, conflicts over water have led to civil unrest, and by enabling individual access to groundwater, we can reduce the risk of such disputes.

Addressing water needs through modern technology is also an investment in future generations. As the global population continues to rise, water demand will only increase. By developing and distributing machines that allow for sustainable water extraction and utilizing modern helicopters for inaccessible regions, I am laying the groundwork for a future in which everyone has the water they need to thrive. It's about creating a lasting solution, one that adapts to the needs of each individual community and prepares the world for the water challenges ahead.

Ultimately, this initiative requires collective effort. Governments, universities, the private sector, and international organizations like the UN must come together to make water access a reality for all. It's a daunting task, but by leveraging modern machine technology and innovative transportation solutions, we can take significant steps toward a world where water is no longer a privilege but a right for everyone. We must act now to make this vision a reality.

Facilitating access to clean and reliable water sources is crucial for the well-being of communities around the world. Water is a fundamental human need, essential for drinking, sanitation, agriculture, and overall health. In many parts of the world, people still struggle to access clean water, which hinders their quality of life. Modern machine technology has the potential to revolutionize how water is sourced and distributed, particularly through innovative solutions like using underground water. If households or communities can tap into underground water from their own compounds, this would alleviate water shortages and drastically improve lives globally.

Using modern machine technology to access underground water could be a game-changer for regions where water is scarce. There are already technologies available that allow people to drill into aquifers and access clean water from below the earth's surface. These machines can be scaled down to be more accessible for individual use, allowing people to install them in their own compounds. By utilizing this resource, individuals can secure their water supply, ensuring that they have clean water for drinking, farming, and other essential needs. This would reduce dependency on unreliable water sources and cut down on long journeys many people currently have to make to find water.

However, some regions may face challenges in accessing underground water due to geological conditions. In such cases, governments can play a pivotal role by stepping in to provide solutions. One potential solution is the use of helicopters specifically designed and manufactured to distribute water in hard-to-reach areas. Government universities, in collaboration with engineering experts, could take the lead in developing such helicopters equipped to transport and distribute water efficiently. This innovative solution would ensure that even those in remote or geologically challenging areas can access the water they need.

In addition to national efforts the United Nations (UN) have a responsibility to address water scarcity on a broader scale. The UN can mobilize resources, expertise, and global cooperation to ensure that modern technology is harnessed to address water needs. By prioritizing water accessibility, the UN can help create a blueprint for sustainable water management, particularly for regions that are hardest hit by water shortages. Ensuring access to water can also help achieve multiple Sustainable Development Goals, including ending poverty and improving health outcomes.

Moreover, the availability of modern technology for water extraction could spark economic growth and development. Access to water would enable communities to engage in agriculture and small-scale industries, creating employment opportunities and reducing poverty. When people have access to water, they can cultivate crops, improve food security, and even develop local businesses related to water-based resources. These economic benefits would lift communities out of poverty and set the stage for long-term development.

Facilitating water access is not just a technical challenge; it also presents an opportunity for educational and research institutions to engage in solving real-world problems. Universities can partner with governments and private organizations to develop new technologies and refine existing ones, making water extraction and distribution more efficient and cost-effective. Involving students and researchers in these initiatives can lead to innovative solutions and ensure that the next generation of engineers and scientists is equipped to address pressing global challenges.

Water access has far-reaching social impacts as well. When people no longer have to worry about finding water for their daily needs, they are freed from the stress and time-consuming efforts involved in securing water. This means children can spend more time in school, and women—who are often the primary water gatherers in many communities—can engage in other productive activities. Improving water access can promote gender equality and provide everyone with the opportunity to live healthier, more productive lives.

For governments and organizations to succeed in addressing water scarcity, they must invest in education and training. People need to be equipped with the knowledge and skills to maintain and use modern water extraction machines. This includes training technicians, engineers, and local leaders to manage and repair the technology. Capacity-building is crucial to ensuring that once modern technologies are deployed, they can be maintained and sustained over the long term.

Facilitating water needs through modern machine technology offers a practical and impactful solution to water scarcity. By empowering people to access underground water from their own compounds or, when necessary, leveraging government intervention with advanced tools like water-transporting helicopters, we can ensure that every community has access to this life-sustaining resource. Collaboration between governments, educational institutions, and the international community—particularly through the leadership of the UN—is key to making this vision a reality. With sustained effort, modern technology can transform lives by providing reliable water access, promoting development, and ensuring a healthier future for all.

Water is the lifeblood of human existence. From sustaining life to driving agriculture and industry, access to water is crucial for every aspect of daily life. In many parts of the world, access to clean water is a constant struggle, a situation that demands urgent attention and innovative solutions. Facilitating water access, particularly by leveraging modern machine technology, could revolutionize the way we meet our water needs. The idea of tapping into underground water sources right from one's own compound holds tremendous potential for transforming lives worldwide. By deploying advanced technologies that make it possible to extract and manage groundwater efficiently, we can bring relief to millions and set a new precedent for how we manage our water resources.

Imagine the impact of a simple machine capable of tapping into underground water reserves on individual properties. Farmers could irrigate their crops without relying on distant water sources, households could access clean drinking water without making long treks, and businesses could flourish in previously water-scarce regions. Such technology could transform arid and semi-arid regions, offering not just survival but the potential for economic growth. The ability to tap into underground water would also minimize the reliance on large-scale infrastructure projects, making water access more personal, localized, and immediate.

There are places where underground water may not be as accessible due to geological constraints. In such cases, innovation does not stop. Governments, in collaboration with universities and technological institutes, can manufacture specialized helicopters designed for water delivery. These helicopters could be outfitted with equipment to extract and transport water to communities that cannot access it on their own. By making water delivery efficient and scalable, these helicopters would allow governments to reach even the most remote or geologically challenging regions. This vision requires investment in technology and infrastructure, but the benefits would be enormous, ensuring that no one is left without the water they need to live and thrive.

The United Nations (UN) plays a vital role in addressing global challenges, and water scarcity is among the most pressing. The UN should prioritize working with member states to develop and implement this kind of technology to ensure that access to clean, reliable water is a reality for everyone. By facilitating partnerships between governments, private industries, and educational institutions, the UN can help create a collaborative platform for technological advancement in water access. This initiative could lead to widespread deployment of water extraction machines and helicopters globally, particularly in regions where water scarcity is a critical issue. Such a concerted effort could save lives and lift entire communities out of the devastating cycle of water poverty.

In many developing nations, especially in rural areas, the water crisis is compounded by limited infrastructure and a lack of technological resources. Implementing modern machine technology that allows people to extract water from their own land would reduce dependence on large-scale, distant water projects and make communities more self-sufficient. Local governments can also play a crucial role by offering subsidies or incentives to households to install these machines. This could be a monumental step toward reducing water inequality, giving even the poorest communities access to life's most basic resource. The process of facilitating water through technology would also stimulate local economies by creating jobs in manufacturing, maintenance, and distribution.

Further, this water-access technology could have environmental benefits. Many traditional methods of water extraction, such as extensive irrigation systems or water transportation, are inefficient and contribute to water waste. Machine technology designed to access underground water would be more sustainable, reducing the need for excessive drilling or construction of reservoirs. Water usage could be monitored and controlled, ensuring that extraction does not deplete local water tables. It would also reduce the need for long-distance transportation of water, cutting down on the environmental impact of fuel consumption and emissions.

Access to water has profound implications for health, especially in regions where waterborne diseases are rampant. The World Health Organization estimates that millions of people die each year from preventable water-related illnesses. Machine technology that provides localized, clean water sources could drastically reduce the occurrence of these diseases. This is not just a matter of convenience; it is a matter of life and death. Improved water access would mean fewer people suffering from diarrheal diseases, cholera, and other infections caused by contaminated water. By ensuring that clean water is available directly from underground sources, communities would be healthier, stronger, and better equipped to contribute to societal progress.

The challenge, of course, is not only about technology but also about equitable distribution. Governments must ensure that water access is not monopolized by wealthier individuals or regions. By partnering with universities, governments can ensure that the necessary expertise is developed locally, fostering innovation that serves the public good rather than private interests. This collaboration could result in the development of technologies that are accessible, affordable, and scalable, ensuring that the benefits of machine-facilitated water access reach every corner of society.

One of the key factors in the success of this initiative is public awareness and education. Communities need to be educated on the importance of sustainable water usage and how to maintain the machines. Schools and universities can play a role in disseminating knowledge about the new technologies, empowering the next generation to carry forward the work of water conservation and access. As the machines are introduced, local training programs can ensure that people know how to operate and maintain them, making the system sustainable in the long term.

Facilitating water access through modern machine technology could be one of the most important innovations of our time. The ability to extract underground water directly from one's property, combined with government-backed helicopter water delivery in difficult areas, has the potential to change lives across the globe. This technological leap would not only address water scarcity but also promote health, economic stability, and environmental sustainability. The UN, governments, and educational institutions must work together to make this vision a reality, ensuring that every person, no matter where they live, has access to the water they need to survive and thrive.

Facilitating access to clean water for human needs is one of the most critical global challenges we face today. Water is an essential element for human survival, agriculture, industry, and overall well-being. Unfortunately, millions of people around the world, particularly in developing regions, still struggle with limited or no access to clean water. Modern technological innovations, specifically in the area of water extraction from underground sources, offer a transformative solution. By leveraging machine technology that allows individuals to access underground water directly from their own compound, we can revolutionize water access and dramatically improve the quality of life for many.

Modern machine technology has the potential to make underground water readily available, even for people living in areas where water scarcity is a daily struggle. A small, efficient machine designed to tap into groundwater reserves on private or communal properties can empower families and communities to become self-sufficient in their water needs. This localized solution would reduce reliance on large-scale water infrastructure projects and offer an immediate and cost-effective way for individuals to meet their daily water requirements. The technology could be designed to be user-friendly, affordable, and sustainable, making it accessible to people in both rural and urban settings.

In regions where underground water is not easily accessible, governments could play a crucial role in facilitating water access. For example, governments could invest in the development of specialized helicopters capable of delivering water to remote areas. These helicopters could be equipped with the necessary technology to extract water from distant underground sources or transport water from areas with abundant water supplies to regions in need. By collaborating with universities and research institutions, governments could ensure that these helicopters are designed and manufactured with state-of-the-art technology, making them both efficient and environmentally friendly.

The integration of government universities in this process is essential for driving innovation and ensuring that water solutions are tailored to the specific needs of different regions. Universities can engage in research and development to create machines that are suited to various geological conditions, making water extraction more efficient. They can also train engineers and technicians to maintain and operate the technology, creating a skilled workforce that can address the issue of water scarcity in a sustainable manner. This collaboration between governments, universities, and the private sector would lead to the creation of a comprehensive water access strategy that meets the needs of all communities.

In addition to government intervention, the United Nations (UN) should take a leadership role in ensuring that water access becomes a global priority. The UN has a long-standing commitment to addressing water scarcity through initiatives such as the Sustainable Development Goals (SDGs), particularly Goal 6, which calls for clean water and sanitation for all. By focusing on the development of machine technology for water extraction and helicopter-based water delivery, the UN can help mobilize international support for this critical issue. This would not only benefit individuals in water-scarce regions but also promote global stability by addressing one of the root causes of conflict and displacement.

Water access is not just a local issue; it has far-reaching implications for global peace and security. Regions that suffer from chronic water shortages are often plagued by social unrest, economic instability, and health crises. By ensuring that people have access to clean, reliable water, we can reduce tensions over water resources and prevent conflicts that arise from competition for scarce resources. Machine technology that allows for local water extraction would provide communities with a sense of security and stability, allowing them to focus on economic development, education, and other areas of growth.

Furthermore, the health benefits of improved water access cannot be overstated. In many parts of the world, people suffer from waterborne diseases due to a lack of clean drinking water. These diseases disproportionately affect children and vulnerable populations, leading to high rates of mortality and chronic illness. By providing clean water through modern technology, we can significantly reduce the prevalence of water-related illnesses and improve public health outcomes. This would have a ripple effect on societies, leading to improved productivity, lower healthcare costs, and overall enhanced quality of life.

From an environmental perspective, machine technology for water extraction also offers a sustainable solution. Traditional methods of water access, such as the construction of large dams and reservoirs, can have significant environmental impacts, including the disruption of ecosystems and the displacement of communities. By contrast, localized water extraction machines would minimize environmental damage by tapping into existing groundwater reserves without the need for large-scale infrastructure projects. This would help preserve natural ecosystems while still meeting the water needs of growing populations.

The economic benefits of facilitating water access through modern technology are equally important. When people have reliable access to water, they can engage in productive activities such as farming, small-scale manufacturing, and other income-generating ventures. This can lift entire communities out of poverty and create opportunities for economic growth and development. In particular, access to water for agriculture would enable farmers to increase crop yields, leading to greater food security and improved livelihoods for rural populations.

Facilitating water access through modern machine technology has the potential to transform lives across the globe. By providing individuals with the tools to extract underground water from their own compounds, we can empower communities to become self-reliant and reduce the burden on centralized water systems. Government collaboration with universities and technological institutions, combined with the leadership of the UN, can make this vision a reality. The development of water-delivery helicopters for hard-to-reach areas further ensures that no one is left behind in the quest for water security. This comprehensive approach to water access would not only address the immediate needs of water-scarce regions but also promote long-term peace, stability, and prosperity for all.

Facilitating access to water is crucial for the survival and development of humanity. In many parts of the world, millions of people still lack reliable access to clean and safe water. Water is not only essential for drinking and sanitation but also for agriculture, industry, and overall economic growth. By embracing modern technology, we can drastically change the way water is sourced, making it easier for people to access underground water directly from their own compounds. The integration of modern machinery designed specifically to tap into underground water reserves holds immense potential to transform lives globally, providing a sustainable solution for water scarcity.

The importance of modern machine technology cannot be overstated when it comes to water needs. Imagine having a machine right in your backyard that can drill and extract underground water with minimal effort. This technology would not only bring water closer to households but also empower communities to manage their water supply independently. Currently, many people rely on distant water sources, walking miles every day, often to unsanitary or depleted wells. Modern machines that make underground water easily accessible can save countless hours, improve hygiene, and support sustainable agriculture, helping to lift communities out of poverty.

For people who encounter issues finding water beneath their own land, governments can step in to provide alternatives. One visionary solution is the development of specialized helicopters that can assist in locating and extracting water in arid or difficult-to-reach areas. Governments can partner with local universities and research institutions to design and manufacture these helicopters, equipped with advanced sensors capable of detecting underground water sources. By deploying such technology, it will be possible to overcome geographical barriers and ensure that water is available in regions where traditional methods of sourcing water fail.

The United Nations should play a leading role in making these ideas a global reality. Access to water is a fundamental human right, and the UN has long been at the forefront of promoting sustainable development goals, including clean water and sanitation for all. By championing modern water extraction technologies, the UN can help mobilize resources and encourage international cooperation. This would not only alleviate water shortages but also contribute to other global challenges such as food security, health, and poverty reduction. The organization has the power to bring governments, research institutions, and the private sector together to develop these innovative solutions.

Water scarcity has long been a challenge, especially in developing countries, where the majority of people are dependent on natural water bodies that are often unreliable or polluted. This technology also has the potential to provide access to clean drinking water in rural areas where building infrastructure such as large pipelines is costly and inefficient. For example, in many African countries, such technology could drastically improve agricultural productivity, which is heavily dependent on water availability.

Helicopter-based water sourcing operations represent an exciting frontier in the quest to provide universal access to water. Governments in cooperation with universities and technological institutes can manufacture helicopters equipped with geo-sensing technology capable of detecting underground water reserves. Once identified, specialized drilling machinery could be deployed directly from the air, thus bypassing the logistical challenges posed by rugged or remote terrain. The helicopter's ability to cover large areas quickly would make it invaluable in large-scale operations, ensuring that no community is left behind, even in the most challenging environments.

The collaboration between governments and universities could also lead to advances in water purification systems that can be coupled with these underground water extraction technologies. Many underground water sources, though abundant, require filtration or treatment to meet safe drinking standards. Government-supported research initiatives could focus on developing portable and affordable water filtration technologies that can be used alongside water extraction systems, ensuring that the water provided to communities is not only plentiful but also clean and safe.

Another key element in solving the water crisis is ensuring that these technological solutions are affordable and scalable. Governments need to subsidize the cost of these machines, making them accessible to the general public. They should work in conjunction with private companies to develop machines that are not only efficient but also cost-effective, ensuring that even the poorest communities can benefit from these innovations. The potential ripple effects of solving water access issues are profound—better health, increased agricultural output, reduced poverty, and enhanced education, all of which contribute to a nation's development.

Governments must also consider the training and education of the population regarding these new technologies. It's essential that individuals know how to use and maintain water extraction machines. Training programs in schools, communities, and agricultural centers can ensure that people are empowered to manage their own water supply. Educated and skilled individuals are better equipped to handle the challenges of water scarcity, and modern technology can help build resilience to water-related crises, ensuring long-term sustainability.

Modern machine technology offers a powerful solution to the world's water challenges. By tapping into underground water sources and leveraging innovations such as helicopter-based water extraction, we can provide sustainable access to water for millions of people. This vision requires the cooperation of governments, universities, international organizations like the UN, and the private sector. With the right investments and political will, water scarcity can become a problem of the past, ensuring that all people, no matter where they live, have access to this precious resource.

Below is repeated version of the above part for the sake of qualification of this investigative water research book publication to see it reaching you in this particular version just to add page number value!

Revolutionizing Water Access Through Modern Technology: A Step Towards Global Change

Investigative Water Research Book

By Meklit Garedew Gebrewold

© 2024 by Meklit Garedew

Cover design by Meklit Garedew Gebrewold

Meklit Garedew Gebrewold's contact: meklitgara91@gmail.com

Introduction

Access to clean and safe water is a fundamental human right, and ensuring its availability can transform lives across the globe. Water is the cornerstone of health, agriculture, and overall well-being, yet millions still struggle to access it. Facilitating water access, especially in areas plagued by scarcity, can break cycles of poverty, improve public health, and elevate the quality of life for countless communities. The ripple effect of accessible water extends to education, economic development, and environmental sustainability, making it a global priority that must not be overlooked.

The United Nations plays a pivotal role in addressing global challenges, and the facilitation of water access should be at the forefront of its agenda. By allocating resources and initiating large-scale projects, the UN can drive significant progress toward ensuring that every person, regardless of location, has reliable access to clean water. This universal water supply requires cooperation and commitment from governments and UN to create sustainable, long-lasting solutions.

Moreover, as humanity looks toward future exploration and the possibility of inhabiting other planets, it is essential to consider how water can be transported and made accessible in extraterrestrial environments. This potential not only highlights the importance of innovation in water technology but also raises the need for global organizations like the UN to take proactive measures in supporting water solutions that transcend Earth.

In addition to global efforts, universities and research institutions must take an active role in addressing water scarcity. Government-funded universities, in particular, have the capacity to develop and implement innovative technologies to tackle this pressing issue. By dedicating time, resources, and research to finding practical, cost-effective solutions, these institutions can spearhead transformative change. Their involvement could lead to groundbreaking discoveries that make water more accessible, especially in regions most affected by shortages.

During my years in medical school, I initiated research on water accessibility after noticing a severe shortage in a specific region of Ethiopia, an area historically known for its water challenges. Every Ethiopian is aware of the significance of this region's long-standing struggle. Even since I was a little kid the way my parents used to manage the water supply for our family is way too unique and I do admire them in such a sincere and lovely way. I do always thank God almighty about them in the name of Jesus Christ for God has given me such awesome plus brave parents! So I was well equipped with so much great wisdoms from my parents then here I am with a priceless fruit in such unpredictable calling of God almighty on my life! Here I am with such a great investigative water research book! With proper dedication and collaboration between academic institutions, governments, and the UN, universal access to water can become a reality.

Revolutionizing Water Access Through Modern Technology: A Step Towards Global Change

Water is a fundamental necessity for all human life, and its scarcity remains a pressing challenge for millions around the world. While we have made significant advancements in various sectors of life, the issue of providing clean and accessible water for everyone still lingers in many parts of the universe. Ensuring that every person has access to adequate water resources is essential not only for survival but also for improving quality of life. Water is critical for agriculture, sanitation, industry, and daily personal use. The question is, how can we harness modern technology to facilitate water needs globally, especially in areas where it remains scarce?

A potential solution lies in utilizing underground water sources from one's own compound. With the advancement of modern machine technology, it is possible to develop equipment that can extract groundwater in a cost-effective and sustainable manner. Imagine a future where households, especially in remote or arid regions, could have personal access to water through specialized technology that taps into underground reserves. This would revolutionize how we think about water supply and usage, eliminating reliance on centralized, and often strained, water infrastructures. For regions that struggle to find surface water, this could be a game-changer.

The beauty of this approach is its ability to empower individuals and communities to take control of their water needs. By creating a small-scale, efficient machine to extract underground water, families could become self-sufficient in their water consumption, reducing the burden on over-exploited natural sources. In times of climate uncertainty, where droughts are becoming more common, this technology could provide a lifeline to families at risk of water insecurity. Furthermore, it offers a sustainable alternative to traditional methods of water sourcing, which often involve lengthy, expensive infrastructure projects that are difficult to maintain.

However, for this to work effectively, I need to ensure that the technology is widely available and accessible to all, especially in low-income areas where water scarcity is most severe. This is where the role of governments becomes crucial. Governments, in collaboration with universities and research institutions, have the capacity to develop, fund, and distribute these modern machines on a national and global scale. Government support is necessary to subsidize the technology, making it affordable for the people who need it most. Collaboration with local academic institutions would provide the technical know-how to develop these machines, creating opportunities for innovation while addressing a critical global need.

In cases where underground water is not accessible in one's own compound or region, a more creative solution is required. One such idea is the use of modern helicopters specifically manufactured to help transport water to remote areas where water wells cannot be established. These helicopters could be equipped with advanced water storage systems and function similarly to air ambulances, providing immediate water relief to those in critical need. Governments, once again, would play a pivotal role in this innovation, developing these specialized helicopters through public-private partnerships and university-driven research.

The role of international bodies such as the United Nations cannot be underestimated in addressing the global water crisis. The UN, with its global influence and resources, should prioritize facilitating water access for every individual. By partnering with nations and supporting the research, development, and deployment of modern water-extraction technologies, the UN can help ensure that everyone, regardless of their location, has access to safe and reliable water. This kind of commitment would align with the UN's Sustainable Development Goals, particularly Goal 6, which aims to ensure the availability and sustainable management of water for all.

The impact of providing water access through modern technology would be profound. It would not only save lives by reducing waterborne diseases and promoting sanitation but also create opportunities for economic growth. In agricultural communities, for example, access to consistent water supplies would enable farmers to increase productivity, ensuring food security. In urban settings, reliable water access would improve living conditions and promote hygiene, contributing to overall public health. This approach would significantly boost the well-being of populations worldwide.

Introducing water-extracting technology at a household level would democratize water access, creating a system that is not reliant on the inefficiencies of government distribution or private monopolies. It would also alleviate political tensions surrounding water rights and distribution, which are common in water-scarce regions. In many cases, conflicts over water have led to civil unrest, and by enabling individual access to groundwater, we can reduce the risk of such disputes.

Addressing water needs through modern technology is also an investment in future generations. As the global population continues to rise, water demand will only increase. By developing and distributing machines that allow for sustainable water extraction and utilizing modern helicopters for inaccessible regions, I am laying the groundwork for a future in which everyone has the water they need to thrive. It's about creating a lasting solution, one that adapts to the needs of each individual community and prepares the world for the water challenges ahead.

Ultimately, this initiative requires collective effort. Governments, universities, the private sector, and international organizations like the UN must come together to make water access a reality for all. It's a daunting task, but by leveraging modern machine technology and innovative transportation solutions, we can take significant steps toward a world where water is no longer a privilege but a right for everyone. We must act now to make this vision a reality.

Facilitating access to clean and reliable water sources is crucial for the well-being of communities around the world. Water is a fundamental human need, essential for drinking, sanitation, agriculture, and overall health. In many parts of the world, people still struggle to access clean water, which hinders their quality of life. Modern machine technology has the potential to revolutionize how water is sourced and distributed, particularly through innovative solutions like using underground water. If households or communities can tap into underground water from their own compounds, this would alleviate water shortages and drastically improve lives globally.

Using modern machine technology to access underground water could be a game-changer for regions where water is scarce. There are already technologies available that allow people to drill into aquifers and access clean water from below the earth's surface. These machines can be scaled down to be more accessible for individual use, allowing people to install them in their own compounds. By utilizing this resource, individuals can secure their water supply, ensuring that they have clean water for drinking, farming, and other essential needs. This would reduce dependency on unreliable water sources and cut down on long journeys many people currently have to make to find water.

However, some regions may face challenges in accessing underground water due to geological conditions. In such cases, governments can play a pivotal role by stepping in to provide solutions. One potential solution is the use of helicopters specifically designed and manufactured to distribute water in hard-to-reach areas. Government universities, in collaboration with engineering experts, could take the lead in developing such helicopters equipped to transport and distribute water efficiently. This innovative solution would ensure that even those in remote or geologically challenging areas can access the water they need.

In addition to national efforts the United Nations (UN) have a responsibility to address water scarcity on a broader scale. The UN can mobilize resources, expertise, and global cooperation to ensure that modern technology is harnessed to address water needs. By prioritizing water accessibility, the UN can help create a blueprint for sustainable water management, particularly for regions that are hardest hit by water shortages. Ensuring access to water can also help achieve multiple Sustainable Development Goals, including ending poverty and improving health outcomes.

Moreover, the availability of modern technology for water extraction could spark economic growth and development. Access to water would enable communities to engage in agriculture and small-scale industries, creating employment opportunities and reducing poverty. When people have access to water, they can cultivate crops, improve food security, and even develop local businesses related to water-based resources. These economic benefits would lift communities out of poverty and set the stage for long-term development.

Facilitating water access is not just a technical challenge; it also presents an opportunity for educational and research institutions to engage in solving real-world problems. Universities can partner with governments and private organizations to develop new technologies and refine existing ones, making water extraction and distribution more efficient and cost-effective. Involving students and researchers in these initiatives can lead to innovative solutions and ensure that the next generation of engineers and scientists is equipped to address pressing global challenges.

Water access has far-reaching social impacts as well. When people no longer have to worry about finding water for their daily needs, they are freed from the stress and time-consuming efforts involved in securing water. This means children can spend more time in school, and women—who are often the primary water gatherers in many communities—can engage in other productive activities. Improving water access can promote gender equality and provide everyone with the opportunity to live healthier, more productive lives.

For governments and organizations to succeed in addressing water scarcity, they must invest in education and training. People need to be equipped with the knowledge and skills to maintain and use modern water extraction machines. This includes training technicians, engineers, and local leaders to manage and repair the technology. Capacity-building is crucial to ensuring that once modern technologies are deployed, they can be maintained and sustained over the long term.

Facilitating water needs through modern machine technology offers a practical and impactful solution to water scarcity. By empowering people to access underground water from their own compounds or, when necessary, leveraging government intervention with advanced tools like water-transporting helicopters, we can ensure that every community has access to this life-sustaining resource. Collaboration between governments, educational institutions, and the international community—particularly through the leadership of the UN—is key to making this vision a reality. With sustained effort, modern technology can transform lives by providing reliable water access, promoting development, and ensuring a healthier future for all.

Water is the lifeblood of human existence. From sustaining life to driving agriculture and industry, access to water is crucial for every aspect of daily life. In many parts of the world, access to clean water is a constant struggle, a situation that demands urgent attention and innovative solutions. Facilitating water access, particularly by leveraging modern machine technology, could revolutionize the way we meet our water needs. The idea of tapping into underground water sources right from one's own compound holds tremendous potential for transforming lives worldwide. By deploying advanced technologies that make it possible to extract and manage groundwater efficiently, we can bring relief to millions and set a new precedent for how we manage our water resources.

Imagine the impact of a simple machine capable of tapping into underground water reserves on individual properties. Farmers could irrigate their crops without relying on distant water sources, households could access clean drinking water without making long treks, and businesses could flourish in previously water-scarce regions. Such technology could transform arid and semi-arid regions, offering not just survival but the potential for economic growth. The ability to tap into underground water would also minimize the reliance on large-scale infrastructure projects, making water access more personal, localized, and immediate.

There are places where underground water may not be as accessible due to geological constraints. In such cases, innovation does not stop. Governments, in collaboration with universities and technological institutes, can manufacture specialized helicopters designed for water delivery. These helicopters could be outfitted with equipment to extract and transport water to communities that cannot access it on their own. By making water delivery efficient and scalable, these helicopters would allow governments to reach even the most remote or geologically challenging regions. This vision requires investment in technology and infrastructure, but the benefits would be enormous, ensuring that no one is left without the water they need to live and thrive.

The United Nations (UN) plays a vital role in addressing global challenges, and water scarcity is among the most pressing. The UN should prioritize working with member states to develop and implement this kind of technology to ensure that access to clean, reliable water is a reality for everyone. By facilitating partnerships between governments, private industries, and educational institutions, the UN can help create a collaborative platform for technological advancement in water access. This initiative could lead to widespread deployment of water extraction machines and helicopters globally, particularly in regions where water scarcity is a critical issue. Such a concerted effort could save lives and lift entire communities out of the devastating cycle of water poverty.

In many developing nations, especially in rural areas, the water crisis is compounded by limited infrastructure and a lack of technological resources. Implementing modern machine technology that allows people to extract water from their own land would reduce dependence on large-scale, distant water projects and make communities more self-sufficient. Local governments can also play a crucial role by offering subsidies or incentives to households to install these machines. This could be a monumental step toward reducing water inequality, giving even the poorest communities access to life's most basic resource. The process of facilitating water through technology would also stimulate local economies by creating jobs in manufacturing, maintenance, and distribution.

Further, this water-access technology could have environmental benefits. Many traditional methods of water extraction, such as extensive irrigation systems or water transportation, are inefficient and contribute to water waste. Machine technology designed to access underground water would be more sustainable, reducing the need for excessive drilling or construction of reservoirs. Water usage could be monitored and controlled, ensuring that extraction does not deplete local water tables. It would also reduce the need for long-distance transportation of water, cutting down on the environmental impact of fuel consumption and emissions.

Access to water has profound implications for health, especially in regions where waterborne diseases are rampant. The World Health Organization estimates that millions of people die each year from preventable water-related illnesses. Machine technology that provides localized, clean water sources could drastically reduce the occurrence of these diseases. This is not just a matter of convenience; it is a matter of life and death. Improved water access would mean fewer people suffering from diarrheal diseases, cholera, and other infections caused by contaminated water. By ensuring that clean water is available directly from underground sources, communities would be healthier, stronger, and better equipped to contribute to societal progress.

The challenge, of course, is not only about technology but also about equitable distribution. Governments must ensure that water access is not monopolized by wealthier individuals or regions. By partnering with universities, governments can ensure that the necessary expertise is developed locally, fostering innovation that serves the public good rather than private interests. This collaboration could result in the development of technologies that are accessible, affordable, and scalable, ensuring that the benefits of machine-facilitated water access reach every corner of society.

One of the key factors in the success of this initiative is public awareness and education. Communities need to be educated on the importance of sustainable water usage and how to maintain the machines. Schools and universities can play a role in disseminating knowledge about the new technologies, empowering the next generation to carry forward the work of water conservation and access. As the machines are introduced, local training programs can ensure that people know how to operate and maintain them, making the system sustainable in the long term.

Facilitating water access through modern machine technology could be one of the most important innovations of our time. The ability to extract underground water directly from one's property, combined with government-backed helicopter water delivery in difficult areas, has the potential to change lives across the globe. This technological leap would not only address water scarcity but also promote health, economic stability, and environmental sustainability. The UN, governments, and educational institutions must work together to make this vision a reality, ensuring that every person, no matter where they live, has access to the water they need to survive and thrive.

Facilitating access to clean water for human needs is one of the most critical global challenges we face today. Water is an essential element for human survival, agriculture, industry, and overall well-being. Unfortunately, millions of people around the world, particularly in developing regions, still struggle with limited or no access to clean water. Modern technological innovations, specifically in the area of water extraction from underground sources, offer a transformative solution. By leveraging machine technology that allows individuals to access underground water directly from their own compound, we can revolutionize water access and dramatically improve the quality of life for many.

Modern machine technology has the potential to make underground water readily available, even for people living in areas where water scarcity is a daily struggle. A small, efficient machine designed to tap into groundwater reserves on private or communal properties can empower families and communities to become self-sufficient in their water needs. This localized solution would reduce reliance on large-scale water infrastructure projects and offer an immediate and cost-effective way for individuals to meet their daily water requirements. The technology could be designed to be user-friendly, affordable, and sustainable, making it accessible to people in both rural and urban settings.

In regions where underground water is not easily accessible, governments could play a crucial role in facilitating water access. For example, governments could invest in the development of specialized helicopters capable of delivering water to remote areas. These helicopters could be equipped with the necessary technology to extract water from distant underground sources or transport water from areas with abundant water supplies to regions in need. By collaborating with universities and research institutions, governments could ensure that these helicopters are designed and manufactured with state-of-the-art technology, making them both efficient and environmentally friendly.

The integration of government universities in this process is essential for driving innovation and ensuring that water solutions are tailored to the specific needs of different regions. Universities can engage in research and development to create machines that are suited to various geological conditions, making water extraction more efficient. They can also train engineers and technicians to maintain and operate the technology, creating a skilled workforce that can address the issue of water scarcity in a sustainable manner. This collaboration between governments, universities, and the private sector would lead to the creation of a comprehensive water access strategy that meets the needs of all communities.

In addition to government intervention, the United Nations (UN) should take a leadership role in ensuring that water access becomes a global priority. The UN has a long-standing commitment to addressing water scarcity through initiatives such as the Sustainable Development Goals (SDGs), particularly Goal 6, which calls for clean water and sanitation for all. By focusing on the development of machine technology for water extraction and helicopter-based water delivery, the UN can help mobilize international support for this critical issue. This would not only benefit individuals in water-scarce regions but also promote global stability by addressing one of the root causes of conflict and displacement.

Water access is not just a local issue; it has far-reaching implications for global peace and security. Regions that suffer from chronic water shortages are often plagued by social unrest, economic instability, and health crises. By ensuring that people have access to clean, reliable water, we can reduce tensions over water resources and prevent conflicts that arise from competition for scarce resources. Machine technology that allows for local water extraction would provide communities with a sense of security and stability, allowing them to focus on economic development, education, and other areas of growth.

Furthermore, the health benefits of improved water access cannot be overstated. In many parts of the world, people suffer from waterborne diseases due to a lack of clean drinking water. These diseases disproportionately affect children and vulnerable populations, leading to high rates of mortality and chronic illness. By providing clean water through modern technology, we can significantly reduce the prevalence of water-related illnesses and improve public health outcomes. This would have a ripple effect on societies, leading to improved productivity, lower healthcare costs, and overall enhanced quality of life.

From an environmental perspective, machine technology for water extraction also offers a sustainable solution. Traditional methods of water access, such as the construction of large dams and reservoirs, can have significant environmental impacts, including the disruption of ecosystems and the displacement of communities. By contrast, localized water extraction machines would minimize environmental damage by tapping into existing groundwater reserves without the need for large-scale infrastructure projects. This would help preserve natural ecosystems while still meeting the water needs of growing populations.

The economic benefits of facilitating water access through modern technology are equally important. When people have reliable access to water, they can engage in productive activities such as farming, small-scale manufacturing, and other income-generating ventures. This can lift entire communities out of poverty and create opportunities for economic growth and development. In particular, access to water for agriculture would enable farmers to increase crop yields, leading to greater food security and improved livelihoods for rural populations.

Facilitating water access through modern machine technology has the potential to transform lives across the globe. By providing individuals with the tools to extract underground water from their own compounds, we can empower communities to become self-reliant and reduce the burden on centralized water systems. Government collaboration with universities and technological institutions, combined with the leadership of the UN, can make this vision a reality. The development of water-delivery helicopters for hard-to-reach areas further ensures that no one is left behind in the quest for water security. This comprehensive approach to water access would not only address the immediate needs of water-scarce regions but also promote long-term peace, stability, and prosperity for all.

Facilitating access to water is crucial for the survival and development of humanity. In many parts of the world, millions of people still lack reliable access to clean and safe water. Water is not only essential for drinking and sanitation but also for agriculture, industry, and overall economic growth. By embracing modern technology, we can drastically change the way water is sourced, making it easier for people to access underground water directly from their own compounds. The integration of modern machinery designed specifically to tap into underground water reserves holds immense potential to transform lives globally, providing a sustainable solution for water scarcity.

The importance of modern machine technology cannot be overstated when it comes to water needs. Imagine having a machine right in your backyard that can drill and extract underground water with minimal effort. This technology would not only bring water closer to households but also empower communities to manage their water supply independently. Currently, many people rely on distant water sources, walking miles every day, often to unsanitary or depleted wells. Modern machines that make underground water easily accessible can save countless hours, improve hygiene, and support sustainable agriculture, helping to lift communities out of poverty.

For people who encounter issues finding water beneath their own land, governments can step in to provide alternatives. One visionary solution is the development of specialized helicopters that can assist in locating and extracting water in arid or difficult-to-reach areas. Governments can partner with local universities and research institutions to design and manufacture these helicopters, equipped with advanced sensors capable of detecting underground water sources. By deploying such technology, it will be possible to overcome geographical barriers and ensure that water is available in regions where traditional methods of sourcing water fail.

The United Nations should play a leading role in making these ideas a global reality. Access to water is a fundamental human right, and the UN has long been at the forefront of promoting sustainable development goals, including clean water and sanitation for all. By championing modern water extraction technologies, the UN can help mobilize resources and encourage international cooperation. This would not only alleviate water shortages but also contribute to other global challenges such as food security, health, and poverty reduction. The organization has the power to bring governments, research institutions, and the private sector together to develop these innovative solutions.

Water scarcity has long been a challenge, especially in developing countries, where the majority of people are dependent on natural water bodies that are often unreliable or polluted. This technology also has the potential to provide access to clean drinking water in rural areas where building infrastructure such as large pipelines is costly and inefficient. For example, in many African countries, such technology could drastically improve agricultural productivity, which is heavily dependent on water availability.

Helicopter-based water sourcing operations represent an exciting frontier in the quest to provide universal access to water. Governments in cooperation with universities and technological institutes can manufacture helicopters equipped with geo-sensing technology capable of detecting underground water reserves. Once identified, specialized drilling machinery could be deployed directly from the air, thus bypassing the logistical challenges posed by rugged or remote terrain. The helicopter's ability to cover large areas quickly would make it invaluable in large-scale operations, ensuring that no community is left behind, even in the most challenging environments.

The collaboration between governments and universities could also lead to advances in water purification systems that can be coupled with these underground water extraction technologies. Many underground water sources, though abundant, require filtration or treatment to meet safe drinking standards. Government-supported research initiatives could focus on developing portable and affordable water filtration technologies that can be used alongside water extraction systems, ensuring that the water provided to communities is not only plentiful but also clean and safe.

Another key element in solving the water crisis is ensuring that these technological solutions are affordable and scalable. Governments need to subsidize the cost of these machines, making them accessible to the general public. They should work in conjunction with private companies to develop machines that are not only efficient but also cost-effective, ensuring that even the poorest communities can benefit from these innovations. The potential ripple effects of solving water access issues are profound—better health, increased agricultural output, reduced poverty, and enhanced education, all of which contribute to a nation's development.

Governments must also consider the training and education of the population regarding these new technologies. It's essential that individuals know how to use and maintain water extraction machines. Training programs in schools, communities, and agricultural centers can ensure that people are empowered to manage their own water supply. Educated and skilled individuals are better equipped to handle the challenges of water scarcity, and modern technology can help build resilience to water-related crises, ensuring long-term sustainability.

Modern machine technology offers a powerful solution to the world's water challenges. By tapping into underground water sources and leveraging innovations such as helicopter-based water extraction, we can provide sustainable access to water for millions of people. This vision requires the cooperation of governments, universities, international organizations like the UN, and the private sector. With the right investments and political will, water scarcity can become a problem of the past, ensuring that all people, no matter where they live, have access to this precious resource.

www.ingramcontent.com/pod-product-compliance
Lightning Source LLC
Chambersburg PA
CBHW051536240526
45471CB00020B/3119